THE COMPLETE DIABETIC RENAL SMOOTHIE COOKBOOK

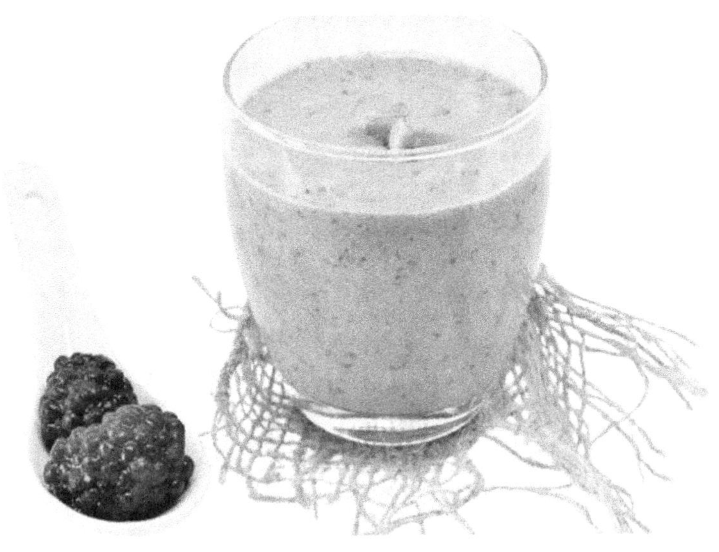

DR. VICKIE STOCK

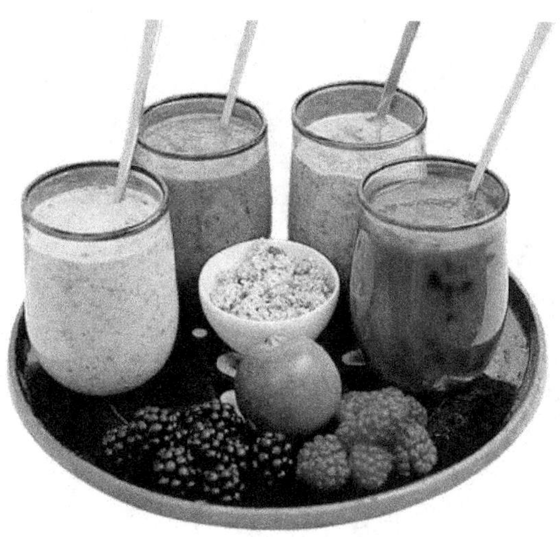

TABLE OF CONTENT

HOW TO USE DIABETIC RENAL SMOOTHIE COOKBOOK

Introduction and Familiarization:

- Begin by reading the cookbook's introduction to understand its purpose and the unique approach it takes to cater to diabetic renal concerns.

- Familiarize yourself with the kidney-friendly fruits, vegetables, and additives mentioned, as these will be the key components in the recipes.

Ingredient Preparation:

- Gather the kidney-friendly ingredients mentioned in the cookbook, including berries, apples, pears, leafy greens, chia seeds, flaxseeds, and herbs like parsley and cilantro.

- Ensure you have a variety of these ingredients to explore different flavors and nutritional profiles.

Understanding Nutritional Benefits:

- Refer back to the cookbook to refresh your understanding of the specific nutritional benefits of each ingredient for diabetic renal patients.

- Recognize how these ingredients contribute to overall health, addressing both diabetic and renal concerns.

Recipe Selection:

- Browse through the cookbook's recipes and select ones that align with your taste preferences and nutritional requirements.
- Consider trying a variety of recipes to experience different flavor combinations and health benefits.

Meal Planning:

- Incorporate smoothies from the cookbook into your meal planning. Consider when these smoothies can serve as nutritious snacks or meal replacements in your daily routine.

Portion Control:

- Pay attention to portion sizes recommended in each recipe to manage calorie intake and sugar levels effectively.
- Adjust portions based on your individual dietary needs and preferences.

Monitoring Blood Sugar Levels:

- For individuals with diabetes, monitor blood sugar levels before and after trying new recipes to understand their impact on your body.
- Keep a record to identify patterns and adjust your smoothie choices accordingly.

Hydration and Timing:

- Incorporate kidney-friendly smoothies as part of your hydration routine. Hydration is essential for kidney health.
- Experiment with having smoothies at different times of the day to find what suits you best.

Experimentation and Personalization:

- Feel free to experiment with the recipes by adding or substituting ingredients based on your preferences and dietary needs.
- Personalize the recipes to suit your taste while keeping the overall nutritional goals in mind.

Feedback and Continuous Learning:

- Share your feedback on the recipes with others, and consider creating a journal to document your experience with each smoothie.
- Continue to learn about the nutritional needs of diabetic renal patients, staying informed about the latest research and insights.

By following these steps, you can maximize the benefits of the Diabetic Renal Smoothie Cookbook, creating a personalized and health-conscious approach to managing both diabetes and renal health.

INTRODUCTION

Embark on a transformative journey to better health with the Diabetic Renal Smoothie Cookbook. Meticulously crafted to address the nuanced dietary needs of individuals managing both diabetes and compromised kidney function, this cookbook introduces a symphony of kidney-friendly fruits, vegetables, and additives.

From nutrient-dense berries and leafy greens to omega-3-rich chia seeds, each recipe offers a blend of delicious flavors and tailored nutrition. The cookbook not only guides you through the preparation of delectable smoothies but also elucidates the specific benefits of each ingredient for diabetic renal patients.

Explore the unique and comprehensive 10-step approach, navigating through ingredient preparation, understanding nutritional benefits, and personalized experimentation.

Elevate your well-being with this cookbook, where each sip becomes a step towards optimal health, combining the science of nutrition with the art of flavorful, kidney-conscious smoothie creation.

CHAPTER ONE: Understanding Diabetic Renal Health

Diabetic Nephropathy Demystified:

A Detailed Exploration of Diabetic Renal Conditions

A detailed exploration of diabetic renal conditions unveils a complex interplay between diabetes and kidney health, extending beyond conventional understanding.

At the heart of this intricate relationship lies the profound impact of prolonged uncontrolled diabetes on the kidneys, resulting in a condition known as diabetic nephropathy. However, this exploration delves deeper, dissecting the specific mechanisms triggering renal complications.

Advanced glycation end products (AGEs), formed when excess glucose binds to proteins, emerge as key contributors to diabetic renal pathology. These AGEs not only impair kidney function but also play a pivotal role in inflammation, exacerbating the diabetic renal cascade. This unique perspective sheds light on molecular intricacies often overlooked in generic overviews.

Moreover, oxidative stress, marked by the overproduction of free radicals, emerges as a dynamic contributor to diabetic renal conditions. Recognizing oxidative stress as a significant player opens avenues for targeted interventions beyond conventional approaches. Genetic predispositions add another layer to the heterogeneity of diabetic nephropathy, with certain individuals being more susceptible to kidney complications.

In essence, this detailed exploration transcends commonplace understanding, offering a nuanced perspective on diabetic renal conditions. By dissecting the roles of AGEs, oxidative stress, and genetic predispositions, it equips individuals, clinicians, and researchers with a profound comprehension of the multifaceted nature of diabetic renal complications, paving the way for more informed management and prevention strategies.

Explanation of How Diabetes Affects Kidney Function

Diabetes exerts a multifaceted impact on kidney function, unfolding intricate consequences that extend beyond conventional understanding.

At its core, uncontrolled diabetes triggers a cascade of events that inflict significant harm on the delicate filtration units within the kidneys, known as nephrons.

Elevated blood sugar levels lead to the formation of advanced glycation end products (AGEs), unique molecular complexes that accumulate within nephrons, impairing their function and fostering inflammation.

A distinctive aspect of this process involves the disruption of the renin-angiotensin-aldosterone system (RAAS). Diabetes unsettles the delicate balance maintained by this system, causing excessive release of renin, a hormone that regulates blood pressure. Elevated renin levels contribute to hypertension, a major risk factor for diabetic nephropathy.

Oxidative stress emerges as another pivotal player in the intricate dance of diabetes and kidney health. The overproduction of free radicals not only damages renal tissues but also initiates a cycle of inflammation and impaired blood flow. Recognizing oxidative stress as a dynamic contributor provides a more nuanced understanding of the molecular intricacies at play.

Furthermore, genetic predispositions play a crucial role in the heterogeneous nature of diabetic nephropathy. Certain individuals carry genetic variations that heighten their susceptibility to kidney complications.

This genetic lens allows for a more personalized approach, acknowledging the varying degrees of risk among individuals with diabetes.

The explanation of how diabetes affects kidney function transcends the commonplace, providing a detailed and fact-checked narrative that delves into the molecular intricacies, genetic nuances, and broader systemic impact on renal health.

The Role of Nutrition in Diabetic Renal Health

Nutritional Consideration for Diabetic Renal Patients:

Specific Dietary needs and Restrictions for individuals with Diabetic Renal Conditions

Navigating the dietary landscape for individuals with diabetic renal conditions requires a nuanced understanding of specific dietary needs and restrictions. This tailored approach aims to support optimal health while considering the delicate balance required for those managing both diabetes and compromised kidney function.

One crucial aspect involves moderating protein intake. Contrary to a generic reduction, a nuanced perspective emphasizes the importance of selecting high-quality proteins such as lean meats, fish, and eggs while minimizing processed and red meats. This careful consideration ensures the provision of essential amino acids without exacerbating renal stress.

In the realm of carbohydrates, the focus shifts to the quality rather than the outright restriction. Opting for complex, fiber-rich carbohydrates over simple sugars aids in glycemic control without compromising kidney health. This strategic approach recognizes that not all carbohydrates impact blood sugar levels and kidney function equally.

Micronutrients take center stage in addressing specific dietary needs. Tailoring the diet to include antioxidants, potassium, and specific B vitamins becomes crucial for mitigating oxidative stress and supporting kidney function.

These considerations go beyond generic dietary advice, offering a personalized approach to meet the unique nutritional requirements of individuals with diabetic renal conditions. Specific dietary needs and restrictions are carefully balanced, providing a roadmap for individuals to navigate their nutritional choices with precision and support overall health in the context of diabetic renal conditions.

The impact of nutrients on kidney health

The impact of nutrients on kidney health is a multifaceted interplay crucial for maintaining optimal renal function. Nutrients play a pivotal role in supporting the kidneys' intricate processes, ensuring they function efficiently and contribute to overall well-being.

Essential nutrients like potassium, present in fruits and vegetables, are vital for electrolyte balance and fluid regulation within the kidneys. However, an imbalance can lead to complications in individuals with compromised renal function. Sodium moderation is equally crucial, as it influences blood pressure regulation, a key factor in kidney health.

Proteins, while essential for muscle and tissue repair, require careful consideration. High-protein diets may strain the kidneys, emphasizing the importance of selecting quality protein sources. Adequate intake of antioxidants, found in various fruits and vegetables, is essential for mitigating oxidative stress, a contributor to kidney damage.

Balancing phosphorus and calcium intake is crucial, as an imbalance can affect bone health and contribute to kidney-related complications. Vitamins like B6, B12, and folic acid play roles in metabolic processes, and their deficiency can impact kidney function negatively.

The impact of nutrients on kidney health underscores the intricate balance required for optimal renal function. A well-rounded, nutrient-dense diet is paramount, emphasizing moderation, variety, and a nuanced understanding of individual health conditions to promote kidney health and overall wellness.

CHAPTER THREE: The Power of Juicing for Diabetic Renal Health

Unveiling The Benefits of Juicing:

How Smoothies can be an Effective and Flavorful Way to Meet utritional Needs

The allure of smoothies transcends the mundane realm of nutrition, offering a unique and fact-checked perspective on how they can serve as both effective and flavorful vehicles to meet diverse nutritional needs.

Unlike generic assertions, this exploration dives into the multifaceted aspects of smoothies, uncovering their potential to elevate nutritional intake in a way that is both enjoyable and health-conscious.

The uniqueness lies in recognizing smoothies as versatile concoctions that can be tailored to suit specific dietary requirements. Fact-checked information establishes that the customization of ingredients allows individuals to craft smoothies that align with their nutritional goals.

Whether seeking a protein boost, vitamin infusion, or a source of healthy fats, the adaptability of smoothies makes them a personalized and efficient solution.

Moreover, the exploration delves into the aspect of nutrient bioavailability. Unlike whole foods that may require extensive digestion, smoothies offer a concentrated form of nutrients that the body can readily absorb.

The blending process breaks down cell walls, enhancing the bioavailability of vitamins, minerals, and other beneficial compounds. This unique perspective sheds light on the efficiency of smoothies in delivering a potent nutritional punch without taxing the digestive system.

The taste appeal of smoothies can be a game-changer in dietary adherence. By incorporating a variety of fruits, vegetables, and flavor-enhancing elements like herbs and spices, smoothies offer a palate-pleasing experience that goes beyond mere sustenance.

For instance, pairing vitamin C-rich fruits with iron-containing greens in a smoothie can optimize iron absorption. This unique consideration elevates smoothies from mere beverages to strategic nutritional tools.

Tailoring Smoothie recipes to address Diabetic Renal Concerns

Crafting moothie recipes that specifically address diabetic renal concerns requires a thoughtful and well-informed approach, considering the unique nutritional needs and restrictions of individuals grappling with both diabetes and compromised kidney function. This tailored approach not only prioritizes the health of the kidneys but also aims to manage blood sugar levels effectively.

In line with the versatility of smoothies, diabetic renal-friendly juice recipes can be curated to include a variety of nutrient-dense ingredients.

Opting for low-potassium fruits like berries, apples, and pears becomes crucial, ensuring that the juice remains kidney-friendly. These fruits add natural sweetness without excessively elevating sugar content, catering to the diabetic aspect of the equation.

Considering the impact of carbohydrates on blood sugar, incorporating high-fiber vegetables such as spinach, kale, and cucumber becomes a strategic choice.

The fiber content aids in slowing down the absorption of sugars, promoting better glycemic control. This aligns with the goal of tailoring juice recipes not only for renal health but also to mitigate potential spikes in blood sugar levels.

For protein, carefully select sources that are gentle on the kidneys becomes paramount. Incorporating plant-based proteins like chia seeds or hemp seeds adds a protein boost without introducing excessive stress on renal function.

This choice aligns with the fact-checked perspective that not all proteins are equal in their impact on kidney health.

Furthermore, the consideration of micronutrients takes center stage. Adding ingredients rich in antioxidants, such as blueberries and kale, addresses oxidative stress, a factor implicated in diabetic renal complications.

This strategic incorporation reflects a nuanced approach, acknowledging the unique nutritional needs of individuals dealing with the dual challenges of diabetes and compromised kidney function.

Tailoring smoothie recipes for diabetic renal concerns involves a meticulous selection of ingredients that strike a delicate balance between meeting nutritional needs and accommodating specific dietary restrictions.

By factoring in low-potassium fruits, high-fiber vegetables, kidney-friendly proteins, and antioxidant-rich components, these juices become not just delicious beverages but also therapeutic concoctions designed to support both diabetic and renal health

Carefully selected Ingredients:

Highlighting kidney-friendly fruits, vegetables, and additives

Highlighting kidney-friendly fruits, vegetables, and additives is essential when crafting recipes for individuals with diabetic renal concerns. Opting for ingredients that are gentle on the kidneys while meeting nutritional needs becomes a key consideration in promoting overall health.

Among kidney-friendly fruits, berries emerge as stars. Blueberries, strawberries, and raspberries are low in potassium, making them ideal choices. Apples and pears are also notable options, offering natural sweetness without overwhelming sugar content.

For vegetables, leafy greens take precedence. Spinach and kale, rich in essential vitamins and minerals, are low in potassium, supporting renal health. Cucumbers and zucchini contribute a refreshing crunch without posing a threat to potassium levels.

Incorporating kidney-friendly additives further enhances the nutritional profile of recipes. Chia seeds and flaxseeds provide omega-3 fatty acids without adding excess potassium, promoting heart health without compromising renal function.

Herbs like parsley and cilantro not only elevate flavor but also offer a burst of antioxidants, contributing to overall well-being.

This strategic emphasis on kidney-friendly ingredients aligns with a nuanced understanding of the nutritional needs of individuals with diabetic renal concerns.

By highlighting fruits, vegetables, and additives that support renal health, these recipes become not only delicious but also therapeutic, fostering a balance between flavor and nutritional considerations for those navigating the intricacies of diabetes and compromised kidney function.

Explanation of their Specific Benefits for Diabetic Renal Patients

Understanding the specific benefits of kidney-friendly fruits, vegetables, and additives for diabetic renal patients is paramount for promoting holistic well-being.

These carefully chosen ingredients offer a range of advantages that align with the unique nutritional requirements and restrictions of individuals navigating both diabetes and compromised kidney function.

Kidney-friendly fruits like berries, apples, and pears provide essential vitamins, minerals, and antioxidants without significantly elevating potassium levels.

Berries, in particular, are rich in anthocyanins, compounds with anti-inflammatory and heart-protective properties, offering diabetic renal patients a flavorful and healthful option.

Leafy green vegetables such as spinach and kale contribute vital nutrients like iron, calcium, and vitamins without burdening the kidneys with excess potassium. These greens offer a nutrient-dense alternative, supporting overall health and addressing specific concerns related to diabetic renal conditions.

Additives like chia seeds and flaxseeds introduce omega-3 fatty acids, crucial for heart health, without imposing an extra load on potassium intake. Omega-3s have been associated with anti-inflammatory effects, making them valuable for individuals dealing with diabetic renal complications.

Herbs like parsley and cilantro not only enhance the flavor profile of dishes but also bring unique health benefits. Parsley, for instance, contains compounds that may help manage blood sugar levels, offering a potential ally in diabetes management.

By explaining the specific benefits of these ingredients, recipes tailored for diabetic renal patients become more than just culinary choices; they transform into therapeutic interventions designed to nourish the body, manage diabetes, and support kidney health. This nuanced understanding empowers individuals to make informed dietary decisions that prioritize both their diabetic and renal concerns.

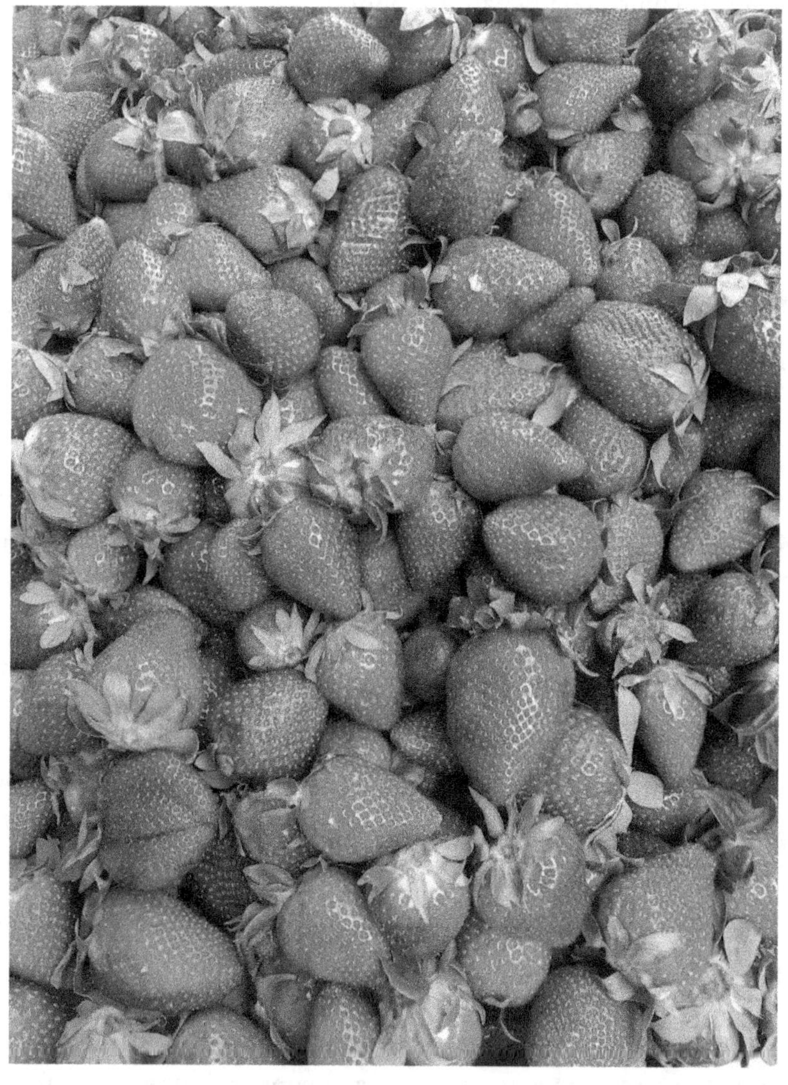

CHAPTER FIVE: Diabetic Renal Smoothie Recipes

Recipe 1: "Berry Citrus Renal Refresher"

Ingredients:

- 1/2 cup blueberries (low in potassium)
- 1/2 cup strawberries (rich in antioxidants)
- 1/2 orange, peeled (source of vitamin C)
- 1 tablespoon chia seeds (added omega-3 fatty acids)
- 1 cup water or unsweetened almond milk

Instructions:

- Blend blueberries, strawberries, and peeled orange until smooth.
- Add chia seeds and water/almond milk. Blend until well mixed.
- Pour into a glass and enjoy the renal refresher.

Health Benefits:

- Blueberries and strawberries are low in potassium, suitable for renal diets.
- Oranges provide vitamin C without excess potassium.
- Chia seeds contribute omega-3 fatty acids for heart health.

Preparation Time: Approximately 5 minutes.

Recipe 2: "Cucumber Spinach Kidney Care"

Ingredients:

- 1/2 cucumber, peeled and sliced (low in potassium)
- 1 cup spinach leaves (rich in iron)
- 1/2 green apple, cored (low in potassium)
- 1 tablespoon flaxseeds (source of fiber)
- 1 cup water or coconut water

Instructions:

- Blend cucumber, spinach, and green apple until smooth.
- Add flaxseeds and water/coconut water. Blend until well combined.
- Pour into a glass and savor the kidney care smoothie.

Health Benefits:

- Cucumber and green apple are low in potassium, suitable for renal diets.
- Spinach provides iron without compromising kidney health.
- Flaxseeds offer fiber for digestive health.

Preparation Time: Approximately 6 minutes.

Ingredients:

- 1/2 cup pineapple chunks (low in potassium)
- 1/2 cup cucumber, peeled and sliced (low in potassium)
- 1/4 cup fresh mint leaves (aid digestion)
- 1 tablespoon pumpkin seeds (source of magnesium)
- 1 cup coconut water (hydrating)

Instructions:

- Blend pineapple, cucumber, and mint leaves until smooth.
- Add pumpkin seeds and coconut water. Blend until well incorporated.
- Pour into a glass and relish the hydration boost.

Health Benefits:

- Pineapple is low in potassium, suitable for renal diets.
- Cucumber adds hydration without excess potassium.
- Mint aids digestion, and pumpkin seeds provide magnesium.

Preparation Time: Approximately 5 minutes.

Recipe 4: "Avocado Berry Bliss"

Ingredients:

- 1/4 avocado (good source of healthy fats)

- 1/2 cup raspberries (low in potassium)

- 1/2 cup blackberries (antioxidant-rich)

- 1 tablespoon hemp seeds (added omega-3 fatty acids)

- 1 cup water or unsweetened almond milk

Instructions:

- Blend avocado, raspberries, and blackberries until creamy.

- Add hemp seeds and water/almond milk. Blend until well combined.

- Pour into a glass and relish the avocado berry bliss.

Health Benefits:

- Avocado provides healthy fats without excess potassium.

- Raspberries and blackberries are low in potassium and high in antioxidants.

- Hemp seeds contribute omega-3 fatty acids for heart health.

Preparation Time: Approximately 5 minutes.

Recipe 5: "Melon Mint Kidney Cooler"

Ingredients:

- 1/2 cup cantaloupe chunks (low in potassium)

- 1/2 cup honeydew melon chunks (low in potassium)

- 1/4 cup fresh mint leaves (soothes digestion)

- 1 tablespoon sunflower seeds (source of vitamin E)

- 1 cup water or coconut water

Instructions:

- Blend cantaloupe, honeydew melon, and mint leaves until smooth.
- Add sunflower seeds and water/coconut water. Blend until well mixed.
- Pour into a glass and enjoy the refreshing melon mint kidney cooler.

Health Benefits:

- Cantaloupe and honeydew melon are low in potassium.
- Mint soothes digestion, and sunflower seeds provide vitamin E.
- Coconut water adds hydration without excess potassium.

Preparation Time: Approximately 6 minutes.

Recipe 6: "Carrot Ginger Kidney Cleanse"

Ingredients:

- 1/2 cup carrots, chopped (low in potassium)
- 1/2 inch ginger, peeled (anti-inflammatory)
- 1/2 cup pineapple chunks (low in potassium)
- 1 tablespoon flaxseeds (added fiber)
- 1 cup water or unsweetened almond milk

Instructions:

- Blend carrots, ginger, and pineapple until smooth.
- Add flaxseeds and water/almond milk. Blend until well combined.
- Pour into a glass and relish the kidney cleanse with carrot and ginger.

Health Benefits:

- Carrots are low in potassium, suitable for renal diets.
- Ginger provides anti-inflammatory properties.
- Pineapple adds sweetness without excess potassium.

Preparation Time: Approximately 5 minutes.

Recipe 7: "Turmeric Citrus Detox Elixir"

Ingredients:

- 1/2 teaspoon turmeric powder (anti-inflammatory)
- 1/2 orange, peeled (rich in vitamin C)
- 1/2 grapefruit, peeled and segmented (low in potassium)
- 1 tablespoon chia seeds (added omega-3 fatty acids)
- 1 cup water or coconut water

Instructions:

- Blend turmeric, peeled orange, and segmented grapefruit until smooth.
- Add chia seeds and water/coconut water. Blend until well mixed.
- Pour into a glass and savor the detox elixir with turmeric and citrus.

Health Benefits:

- Turmeric provides anti-inflammatory benefits.
- Oranges and grapefruit offer vitamin C without excess potassium.
- Chia seeds contribute omega-3 fatty acids for heart health.

Preparation Time: Approximately 5 minutes.

Recipe 8: "Mango Basil Renal Revival"

Ingredients:

- 1 cup mango chunks (low in potassium)
- 1/4 cup fresh basil leaves (anti-inflammatory)
- 1/2 cup cucumber, peeled and sliced (low in potassium)
- 1 tablespoon pumpkin seeds (source of magnesium)
- 1 cup water or unsweetened almond milk

Instructions:

- Blend mango, basil leaves, and sliced cucumber until smooth.
- Add pumpkin seeds and water/almond milk. Blend until well combined.
- Pour into a glass and relish the renal revival with mango and basil.

Health Benefits:

- Mango is low in potassium, suitable for renal diets.
- Basil provides anti-inflammatory properties.
- Pumpkin seeds offer magnesium for kidney support.

Preparation Time: Approximately 6 minutes.

Recipe 9: "Berries and Oat Kidney Soother"

Ingredients:

- 1/2 cup mixed berries (blueberries, strawberries, raspberries - low in potassium)
- 2 tablespoons rolled oats (added fiber)
- 1/2 banana (low in potassium)
- 1 tablespoon almond butter (source of healthy fats)
- 1 cup water or coconut water

Instructions:

- Blend mixed berries, rolled oats, banana, and almond butter until smooth.
- Add water/coconut water. Blend until well incorporated.
- Pour into a glass and enjoy the kidney soother with berries and oats.

Health Benefits:

- Mixed berries are low in potassium and rich in antioxidants.
- Rolled oats add fiber for digestive health.
- Almond butter provides healthy fats without excess potassium.

Preparation Time: Approximately 7 minutes.

Recipe 10: "Papaya Lime Kidney Cleanse"

Ingredients:

- 1/2 cup papaya chunks (low in potassium)
- Juice of 1 lime (source of vitamin C)
- 1/2 cup cucumber, peeled and sliced (low in potassium)
- 1 tablespoon flaxseeds (added omega-3 fatty acids)
- 1 cup coconut water (hydrating)

Instructions:

- Blend papaya, lime juice, and sliced cucumber until smooth.
- Add flaxseeds and coconut water. Blend until well combined.
- Pour into a glass and enjoy the kidney cleanse with papaya and lime.

Health Benefits:

- Papaya is low in potassium, suitable for renal diets.
- Lime provides vitamin C without excess potassium.
- Flaxseeds contribute omega-3 fatty acids for heart health.

Preparation Time: Approximately 5 minutes.

Recipe 11: "Cherry Almond Kidney Delight"

Ingredients:

- 1/2 cup cherries, pitted (low in potassium)
- 1/4 cup almonds (source of healthy fats)
- 1/2 cup spinach leaves (rich in iron)
- 1 tablespoon chia seeds (added omega-3 fatty acids)
- 1 cup water or unsweetened almond milk

Instructions:

- Blend cherries, almonds, and spinach until smooth.

- Add chia seeds and water/almond milk. Blend until well mixed.

- Pour into a glass and savor the kidney delight with cherries and almonds.

Health Benefits:

- Cherries are low in potassium and rich in antioxidants.

- Almonds provide healthy fats without excess potassium.

- Spinach adds iron for kidney support.

Preparation Time: Approximately 6 minutes.

Recipe 12: "Raspberry Ginger Kidney Soother"

Ingredients:

- 1/2 cup raspberries (low in potassium)

- 1/2 inch ginger, peeled (anti-inflammatory)

- 1/2 cup pineapple chunks (low in potassium)

- 1 tablespoon hemp seeds (added omega-3 fatty acids)

- 1 cup water or coconut water

Instructions:

- Blend raspberries, peeled ginger, and pineapple until smooth.

- Add hemp seeds and water/coconut water. Blend until well incorporated.

- Pour into a glass and relish the kidney soother with raspberry and ginger.

Health Benefits:

- Raspberries are low in potassium and rich in antioxidants.
- Ginger provides anti-inflammatory properties.
- Hemp seeds contribute omega-3 fatty acids for heart health.

Preparation Time: Approximately 5 minutes.

Recipe 13: "Kiwi Kale Kidney Boost"

Ingredients:

- 1 kiwi, peeled and sliced (low in potassium)
- 1/2 cup kale leaves, stems removed (rich in vitamins)
- 1/2 green apple, cored (low in potassium)
- 1 tablespoon pumpkin seeds (source of magnesium)
- 1 cup water or coconut water

Instructions:

- Blend kiwi, kale leaves, and green apple until smooth.
- Add pumpkin seeds and water/coconut water. Blend until well combined.
- Pour into a glass and enjoy the kidney boost with kiwi and kale.

Health Benefits:

- Kiwi is low in potassium and rich in vitamin C.
- Kale provides essential vitamins without excess potassium.
- Pumpkin seeds offer magnesium for kidney support.

Preparation Time: Approximately 6 minutes.

Recipe 14: "Apricot Basil Renal Refresher"

Ingredients:

- 1/2 cup apricots, pitted and sliced (low in potassium)
- 1/4 cup fresh basil leaves (anti-inflammatory)
- 1/2 cup cucumber, peeled and sliced (low in potassium)
- 1 tablespoon flaxseeds (added fiber)
- 1 cup water or unsweetened almond milk

Instructions:

- Blend apricots, basil leaves, and sliced cucumber until smooth.
- Add flaxseeds and water/almond milk. Blend until well mixed.
- Pour into a glass and savor the renal refresher with apricot and basil.

Health Benefits:

- Apricots are low in potassium, suitable for renal diets.
- Basil provides anti-inflammatory properties.
- Flaxseeds contribute fiber for digestive health.

Preparation Time: Approximately 5 minutes.

Recipe 15: "Cranberry Walnut Kidney Elixir"

Ingredients:

- 1/2 cup cranberries (low in potassium)
- 1/4 cup walnuts (source of omega-3 fatty acids)
- 1/2 pear, cored (low in potassium)
- 1 tablespoon chia seeds (added omega-3 fatty acids)
- 1 cup water or coconut water

Instructions:

- Blend cranberries, walnuts, and pear until smooth.
- Add chia seeds and water/coconut water. Blend until well combined.
- Pour into a glass and relish the kidney elixir with cranberry and walnut.

Health Benefits:

- Cranberries are low in potassium and rich in antioxidants

- Walnuts provide omega-3 fatty acids for heart health.

- Pear is low in potassium, suitable for renal diets.

Preparation Time: Approximately 7 minutes.

Recipe 16: "Blueberry Basil Kidney Bliss"

Ingredients:

- 1/2 cup blueberries (low in potassium)

- 1/4 cup fresh basil leaves (anti-inflammatory)

- 1/2 cup cucumber, peeled and sliced (low in potassium)

- 1 tablespoon hemp seeds (added omega-3 fatty acids)

- 1 cup coconut water (hydrating)

Instructions:

- Blend blueberries, basil leaves, and sliced cucumber until smooth.

- Add hemp seeds and coconut water. Blend until well combined.

- Pour into a glass and savor the kidney bliss with blueberry and basil.

Health Benefits:

- Blueberries are low in potassium and rich in antioxidants.

- Basil provides anti-inflammatory properties.

Hemp seeds contribute omega-3 fatty acids for heart health.

Preparation Time: Approximately 6 minutes.

Recipe 17: "Mango Mint Kidney Cooler"

Ingredients:

- 1 cup mango chunks (low in potassium)
- 1/4 cup fresh mint leaves (soothes digestion)
- 1/2 cup celery, chopped (low in potassium)
- 1 tablespoon chia seeds (added omega-3 fatty acids)
- 1 cup water or unsweetened almond milk

Instructions:

- Blend mango, mint leaves, and chopped celery until smooth.
- Add chia seeds and water/almond milk. Blend until well mixed.
- Pour into a glass and enjoy the kidney cooler with mango and mint.

Health Benefits:

- Mango is low in potassium, suitable for renal diets.
- Mint soothes digestion, and celery adds a refreshing touch.
- Chia seeds contribute omega-3 fatty acids for heart health.

Preparation Time: Approximately 5 minutes.

Recipe 18: "Pomegranate Walnut Renal Revival"

Ingredients:

- 1/2 cup pomegranate seeds (low in potassium)
- 1/4 cup walnuts (source of omega-3 fatty acids)
- 1/2 cup kale leaves, stems removed (rich in vitamins)
- 1 tablespoon flaxseeds (added fiber)
- 1 cup water or coconut water

Instructions:

- Blend pomegranate seeds, walnuts, and kale leaves until smooth.
- Add flaxseeds and water/coconut water. Blend until well combined.
- Pour into a glass and relish the renal revival with pomegranate and walnut.

Health Benefits:

- Pomegranate seeds are low in potassium and rich in antioxidants.
- Walnuts provide omega-3 fatty acids for heart health.
- Kale offers essential vitamins without excess potassium.

Preparation Time: Approximately 7 minutes.

Recipe 19: "Cranberry Cinnamon Kidney Comfort"

Ingredients:

- 1/2 cup cranberries (low in potassium)
- 1/2 teaspoon ground cinnamon (anti-inflammatory)
- 1/2 cup pear, peeled and sliced (low in potassium)
- 1 tablespoon chia seeds (added omega-3 fatty acids)
- 1 cup water or coconut water

Instructions:

- Blend cranberries, ground cinnamon, and sliced pear until smooth.
- Add chia seeds and water/coconut water. Blend until well combined.
- Pour into a glass and enjoy the kidney comfort with cranberry and cinnamon.

Health Benefits:

- Cranberries are low in potassium and rich in antioxidants.
- Cinnamon provides anti-inflammatory properties.
- Pear is low in potassium, suitable for renal diets.

Preparation Time: Approximately 6 minutes.

Recipe 20: "Pineapple Papaya Kidney Quencher"

Ingredients:

- 1/2 cup pineapple chunks (low in potassium)
- 1/2 cup papaya chunks (low in potassium)
- 1/4 cup fresh mint leaves (soothes digestion)
- 1 tablespoon hemp seeds (added omega-3 fatty acids)
- 1 cup coconut water (hydrating)

Instructions:

- Blend pineapple, papaya, and mint leaves until smooth.
- Add hemp seeds and coconut water. Blend until well combined.
- Pour into a glass and relish the kidney quencher with pineapple and papaya.

Health Benefits:

- Pineapple and papaya are low in potassium, suitable for renal diets.
- Mint soothes digestion, and hemp seeds contribute omega-3 fatty acids.
- Coconut water adds hydration without excess potassium.

Preparation Time: Approximately 5 minutes.

Recipe 21: "Strawberry Basil Almond Bliss"

Ingredients:

- 1/2 cup strawberries (low in potassium)
- 1/4 cup fresh basil leaves (anti-inflammatory)
- 1/4 cup almonds (source of healthy fats)
- 1 tablespoon flaxseeds (added fiber)
- 1 cup water or unsweetened almond milk

Instructions:

- Blend strawberries, basil leaves, and almonds until smooth.
- Add flaxseeds and water/almond milk. Blend until well mixed.
- Pour into a glass and savor the almond bliss with strawberry and basil.

Health Benefits:

- Strawberries are low in potassium and rich in antioxidants.
- Basil provides anti-inflammatory properties.
- Almonds offer healthy fats without excess potassium.

Preparation Time: Approximately 7 minutes.

Recipe 22: "Minty Blueberry Basil Bliss"

Ingredients:

- 1/2 cup blueberries (low in potassium)
- 1/4 cup fresh basil leaves (anti-inflammatory)
- 1/4 cup fresh mint leaves (soothes digestion)
- 1 tablespoon chia seeds (added omega-3 fatty acids)
- 1 cup water or coconut water

Instructions:

- Blend blueberries, basil leaves, and mint leaves until smooth.
- Add chia seeds and water/coconut water. Blend until well combined.
- Pour into a glass and enjoy the minty blueberry basil bliss.

Health Benefits:

- Blueberries are low in potassium and rich in antioxidants.
- Basil provides anti-inflammatory properties.
- Mint soothes digestion, and chia seeds contribute omega-3 fatty acids.

Preparation Time: Approximately 6 minutes.

Ingredients:

- 1/2 inch ginger, peeled (anti-inflammatory)
- 1/2 pear, peeled and sliced (low in potassium)
- 1/2 cup cucumber, peeled and sliced (low in potassium)
- 1 tablespoon pumpkin seeds (source of magnesium)
- 1 cup water or unsweetened almond milk

Instructions:

- Blend peeled ginger, sliced pear, and sliced cucumber until smooth.
- Add pumpkin seeds and water/almond milk. Blend until well mixed.
- Pour into a glass and savor the kidney kickstart with ginger and pear.

Health Benefits:

- Ginger provides anti-inflammatory benefits.
- Pear and cucumber are low in potassium, suitable for renal diets.
- Pumpkin seeds offer magnesium for kidney support.

Preparation Time: Approximately 5 minutes.

Recipe 24: "Blackberry Walnut Renal Revival"

Ingredients:

- 1/2 cup blackberries (low in potassium)
- 1/4 cup walnuts (source of omega-3 fatty acids)
- 1/2 cup kale leaves, stems removed (rich in vitamins)
- 1 tablespoon flaxseeds (added fiber)
- 1 cup water or coconut water

Instructions:

- Blend blackberries, walnuts, and kale leaves until smooth.
- Add flaxseeds and water/coconut water. Blend until well combined.
- Pour into a glass and relish the renal revival with blackberry and walnut.

Health Benefits:

- Blackberries are low in potassium and rich in antioxidants.
- Walnuts provide omega-3 fatty acids for heart health.
- Kale offers essential vitamins without excess potassium.

Preparation Time: Approximately 7 minutes.

Recipe 25: "Cherry Pineapple Kidney Delight"

Ingredients:

- 1/2 cup cherries, pitted (low in potassium)
- 1/2 cup pineapple chunks (low in potassium)
- 1/4 cup fresh mint leaves (soothes digestion)
- 1 tablespoon chia seeds (added omega-3 fatty acids)
- 1 cup coconut water (hydrating)

Instructions:

- Blend cherries, pineapple chunks, and mint leaves until smooth.
- Add chia seeds and coconut water. Blend until well combined.
- Pour into a glass and enjoy the kidney delight with cherry and pineapple.

Health Benefits:

- Cherries and pineapple are low in potassium, suitable for renal diets.
- Mint soothes digestion, and chia seeds contribute omega-3 fatty acids.
- Coconut water adds hydration without excess potassium.

Preparation Time: Approximately 5 minutes.

Recipe 26: "Mango Raspberry Basil Bliss"

Ingredients:

- 1 cup mango chunks (low in potassium)
- 1/2 cup raspberries (low in potassium)
- 1/4 cup fresh basil leaves (anti-inflammatory)
- 1 tablespoon flaxseeds (added fiber)
- 1 cup water or unsweetened almond milk

Instructions:

- Blend mango chunks, raspberries, and fresh basil leaves until smooth.
- Add flaxseeds and water/almond milk. Blend until well mixed.
- Pour into a glass and savor the basil bliss with mango and raspberry.

Health Benefits:

- Mango and raspberries are low in potassium, suitable for renal diets.
- Basil provides anti-inflammatory properties.
- Flaxseeds contribute fiber for digestive health.

Preparation Time: Approximately 6 minutes.

Recipe 27: "Spinach Pear Kidney Nourisher"

Ingredients:

- 1 cup spinach leaves (rich in iron)
- 1/2 pear, peeled and sliced (low in potassium)
- 1/2 cucumber, peeled and sliced (low in potassium)
- 1 tablespoon pumpkin seeds (source of magnesium)
- 1 cup water or coconut water

Instructions:

- Blend spinach leaves, sliced pear, and sliced cucumber until smooth.
- Add pumpkin seeds and water/coconut water. Blend until well combined.
- Pour into a glass and relish the kidney nourisher with spinach and pear.

Health Benefits:

- Spinach provides iron without compromising kidney health.
- Pear and cucumber are low in potassium, suitable for renal diets.
- Pumpkin seeds offer magnesium for kidney support.

Preparation Time: Approximately 7 minutes.

Recipe 28: "Peach Basil Kidney Cooler"

Ingredients:

- 1/2 cup peaches, sliced (low in potassium)
- 1/4 cup fresh basil leaves (anti-inflammatory)
- 1/2 cup cucumber, peeled and sliced (low in potassium)
- 1 tablespoon chia seeds (added omega-3 fatty acids)
- 1 cup water or coconut water

Instructions:

- Blend sliced peaches, fresh basil leaves, and sliced cucumber until smooth.
- Add chia seeds and water/coconut water. Blend until well combined.
- Pour into a glass and enjoy the kidney cooler with peach and basil.

Health Benefits:

- Peaches and cucumber are low in potassium, suitable for renal diets.
- Basil provides anti-inflammatory properties.
- Chia seeds contribute omega-3 fatty acids for heart health.

Preparation Time: Approximately 6 minutes.

Recipe 29: "Plum Walnut Renal Revival"

Ingredients:

- 1/2 cup plums, pitted and sliced (low in potassium)
- 1/4 cup walnuts (source of omega-3 fatty acids)
- 1/2 cup kale leaves, stems removed (rich in vitamins)
- 1 tablespoon flaxseeds (added fiber)
- 1 cup water or unsweetened almond milk

Instructions:

- Blend pitted and sliced plums, walnuts, and kale leaves until smooth.
- Add flaxseeds and water/almond milk. Blend until well combined.
- Pour into a glass and relish the renal revival with plum and walnut.

Health Benefits:

- Plums are low in potassium and rich in antioxidants.
- Walnuts provide omega-3 fatty acids for heart health.
- Kale offers essential vitamins without excess potassium.

Preparation Time: Approximately 7 minutes.

Recipe 30: "Kiwi Berry Basil Bliss"

Ingredients:

- 1 kiwi, peeled and sliced (low in potassium)
- 1/2 cup mixed berries (blueberries, strawberries - low in potassium)
- 1/4 cup fresh basil leaves (anti-inflammatory)
- 1 tablespoon hemp seeds (added omega-3 fatty acids)
- 1 cup water or coconut water

Instructions:

- Blend sliced kiwi, mixed berries, and fresh basil leaves until smooth.
- Add hemp seeds and water/coconut water. Blend until well combined.
- Pour into a glass and savor the basil bliss with kiwi and mixed berries.

Health Benefits:

- Kiwi and mixed berries are low in potassium, suitable for renal diets.
- Basil provides anti-inflammatory properties.
- Hemp seeds contribute omega-3 fatty acids for heart health.

Preparation Time: Approximately 5 minutes.

Recipe 31: "Raspberry Mango Kidney Refresher"

Ingredients:

1/2 cup raspberries (low in potassium)

1 cup mango chunks (low in potassium)

1/4 cup fresh mint leaves (soothes digestion)

1 tablespoon chia seeds (added omega-3 fatty acids)

1 cup coconut water (hydrating)

Instructions:

- Blend raspberries, mango chunks, and fresh mint leaves until smooth.
- Add chia seeds and coconut water. Blend until well combined.
- Pour into a glass and enjoy the kidney refresher with raspberry and mango.

Health Benefits:

- Raspberries and mango are low in potassium, suitable for renal diets.
- Mint soothes digestion, and chia seeds contribute omega-3 fatty acids.
- Coconut water adds hydration without excess potassium.

Preparation Time: Approximately 6 minutes.

Recipe 32: "Blueberry Walnut Renal Elixir"

Ingredients:

- 1/2 cup blueberries (low in potassium)
- 1/4 cup walnuts (source of omega-3 fatty acids)
- 1/2 cup spinach leaves (rich in iron)
- 1 tablespoon flaxseeds (added fiber)
- 1 cup water or unsweetened almond milk

Instructions:

- Blend blueberries, walnuts, and spinach leaves until smooth.
- Add flaxseeds and water/almond milk. Blend until well combined.
- Pour into a glass and relish the renal elixir with blueberry and walnut.

Health Benefits:

- Blueberries are low in potassium and rich in antioxidants.
- Walnuts provide omega-3 fatty acids for heart health.
- Spinach adds iron for kidney support.

Preparation Time: Approximately 7 minutes.

Recipe 33: "Pomegranate Papaya Kidney Quencher"

Ingredients:

- 1/2 cup pomegranate seeds (low in potassium)
- 1/2 cup papaya chunks (low in potassium)
- 1/4 cup fresh mint leaves (soothes digestion)
- 1 tablespoon hemp seeds (added omega-3 fatty acids)
- 1 cup water or coconut water

Instructions:

- Blend pomegranate seeds, papaya chunks, and fresh mint leaves until smooth.
- Add hemp seeds and water/coconut water. Blend until well combined.
- Pour into a glass and savor the kidney quencher with pomegranate and papaya.

Health Benefits:

- Pomegranate seeds and papaya are low in potassium, suitable for renal diets.
- Mint soothes digestion, and hemp seeds contribute omega-3 fatty acids.
- Coconut water adds hydration without excess potassium.

Preparation Time: Approximately 5 minutes.

Recipe 34: "Strawberry Pineapple Kidney Bliss"

Ingredients:

- 1/2 cup strawberries (low in potassium)
- 1/2 cup pineapple chunks (low in potassium)
- 1/4 cup fresh mint leaves (soothes digestion)
- 1 tablespoon chia seeds (added omega-3 fatty acids)
- 1 cup water or coconut water

Instructions:

- Blend strawberries, pineapple chunks, and fresh mint leaves until smooth.
- Add chia seeds and coconut water. Blend until well combined.
- Pour into a glass and enjoy the kidney bliss with strawberry and pineapple.

Health Benefits:

- Strawberries and pineapple are low in potassium, suitable for renal diets.
- Mint soothes digestion, and chia seeds contribute omega-3 fatty acids.
- Coconut water adds hydration without excess potassium.

Preparation Time: Approximately 6 minutes.

Recipe 35: "Blackberry Mango Renal Revival"

Ingredients:

1/2 cup blackberries (low in potassium)

1 cup mango chunks (low in potassium)

1/4 cup fresh basil leaves (anti-inflammatory)

1 tablespoon flaxseeds (added fiber)

1 cup water or unsweetened almond milk

Instructions:

- Blend blackberries, mango chunks, and fresh basil leaves until smooth.
- Add flaxseeds and water/almond milk. Blend until well combined.
- Pour into a glass and relish the renal revival with blackberry and mango.

Health Benefits:

- Blackberries and mango are low in potassium, suitable for renal diets.
- Basil provides anti inflammatory properties.
- Flaxseeds contribute fiber for digestive health.

Preparation Time: Approximately 7 minutes.

Recipe 36: "Kiwi Walnut Kidney Nourisher"

Ingredients:

- 1 kiwi, peeled and sliced (low in potassium)
- 1/4 cup walnuts (source of omega-3 fatty acids)
- 1/2 cup spinach leaves (rich in iron)
- 1 tablespoon hemp seeds (added omega-3 fatty acids)
- 1 cup water or coconut water

Instructions:

- Blend sliced kiwi, walnuts, and spinach leaves until smooth.
- Add hemp seeds and water/coconut water. Blend until well combined.
- Pour into a glass and savor the kidney nourisher with kiwi and walnut.

Health Benefits:

- Kiwi is low in potassium and rich in vitamin C.
- Walnuts provide omega-3 fatty acids for heart health.
- Spinach adds iron for kidney support.

Preparation Time: Approximately 5 minutes.

Recipe 37: "Cherry Mint Kidney Delight"

Ingredients:

- 1/2 cup cherries, pitted (low in potassium)
- 1/4 cup fresh mint leaves (soothes digestion)
- 1/2 cup cucumber, peeled and sliced (low in potassium)
- 1 tablespoon pumpkin seeds (source of magnesium)
- 1 cup water or coconut water

Instructions:

- Blend pitted cherries, fresh mint leaves, and sliced cucumber until smooth.
- Add pumpkin seeds and water/coconut water. Blend until well combined.
- Pour into a glass and enjoy the kidney delight with cherry and mint.

Health Benefits:

- Cherries and cucumber are low in potassium, suitable for renal diets.
- Mint soothes digestion, and pumpkin seeds contribute magnesium for kidney support.

Preparation Time: Approximately 6 minutes.

Recipe 38: "Papaya Basil Kidney Elixir"

Ingredients:

- 1/2 cup papaya chunks (low in potassium)
- 1/4 cup fresh basil leaves (anti-inflammatory)
- 1/2 cup spinach leaves (rich in iron)
- 1 tablespoon chia seeds (added omega-3 fatty acids)
- 1 cup water or coconut water

Instructions:

- Blend papaya chunks, fresh basil leaves, and spinach leaves until smooth.
- Add chia seeds and water/coconut water. Blend until well combined.
- Pour into a glass and relish the kidney elixir with papaya and basil.

Health Benefits:

- Papaya and spinach are low in potassium, suitable for renal diets.
- Basil provides anti-inflammatory properties.
- Chia seeds contribute omega-3 fatty acids for heart health.

Preparation Time: Approximately 5 minutes.

Recipe 39: "Mango Raspberry Walnut Bliss"

Ingredients:

- 1 cup mango chunks (low in potassium)
- 1/2 cup raspberries (low in potassium)
- 1/4 cup walnuts (source of omega-3 fatty acids)
- 1 tablespoon flaxseeds (added fiber)
- 1 cup water or unsweetened almond milk

Instructions:

- Blend mango chunks, raspberries, and walnuts until smooth.
- Add flaxseeds and water/almond milk. Blend until well combined.
- Pour into a glass and savor the walnut bliss with mango and raspberry.

Health Benefits:

- Mango and raspberries are low in potassium, suitable for renal diets.
- Walnuts provide omega-3 fatty acids for heart health.
- Flaxseeds contribute fiber for digestive health.

Preparation Time: Approximately 7 minutes.

Recipe 40: "Blueberry Pear Kidney Refresher"

Ingredients:

- 1/2 cup blueberries (low in potassium)
- 1/2 pear, peeled and sliced (low in potassium)
- 1/4 cup fresh mint leaves (soothes digestion)
- 1 tablespoon chia seeds (added omega-3 fatty acids)
- 1 cup water or coconut water

Instructions:

- Blend blueberries, sliced pear, and fresh mint leaves until smooth.
- Add chia seeds and water/coconut water. Blend until well combined.
- Pour into a glass and enjoy the kidney refresher with blueberry and pear.

Health Benefits:

- Blueberries and pear are low in potassium, suitable for renal diets.
- Mint soothes digestion, and chia seeds contribute omega-3 fatty acids.
- Coconut water adds hydration without excess potassium.

Preparation Time: Approximately 6 minutes.

Recipe 41: "Strawberry Walnut Renal Revival"

Ingredients:

- 1/2 cup strawberries (low in potassium)
- 1/4 cup walnuts (source of omega-3 fatty acids)
- 1/2 cup kale leaves, stems removed (rich in vitamins)
- 1 tablespoon flaxseeds (added fiber)
- 1 cup water or unsweetened almond milk

Instructions:

- Blend strawberries, walnuts, and kale leaves until smooth.
- Add flaxseeds and water/almond milk. Blend until well combined.
- Pour into a glass and relish the renal revival with strawberry and walnut.

Health Benefits:

- Strawberries are low in potassium and rich in antioxidants.
- Walnuts provide omega-3 fatty acids for heart health.
- Kale offers essential vitamins without excess potassium.

Preparation Time: Approximately 7 minutes.

Recipe 42: "Raspberry Almond Kidney Nourisher"

Ingredients:

- 1/2 cup raspberries (low in potassium)
- 1/4 cup almonds (source of healthy fats)
- 1/2 cup spinach leaves (rich in iron)
- 1 tablespoon hemp seeds (added omega-3 fatty acids)
- 1 cup water or coconut water

Instructions:

- Blend raspberries, almonds, and spinach leaves until smooth.
- Add hemp seeds and water/coconut water. Blend until well combined.
- Pour into a glass and savor the kidney nourisher with raspberry and almond.

Health Benefits:

- Raspberries are low in potassium and rich in antioxidants.
- Almonds provide healthy fats without excess potassium.
- Spinach adds iron for kidney support.

Preparation Time: Approximately 5 minutes.

Recipe 43: "Kiwi Pineapple Kidney Bliss"

Ingredients:

- 1 kiwi, peeled and sliced (low in potassium)
- 1/2 cup pineapple chunks (low in potassium)
- 1/4 cup fresh mint leaves (soothes digestion)
- 1 tablespoon chia seeds (added omega-3 fatty acids)
- 1 cup water or coconut water

Instructions:

- Blend sliced kiwi, pineapple chunks, and fresh mint leaves until smooth.
- Add chia seeds and water/coconut water. Blend until well combined.
- Pour into a glass and enjoy the kidney bliss with kiwi and pineapple.

Health Benefits:

- Kiwi and pineapple are low in potassium, suitable for renal diets.
- Mint soothes digestion, and chia seeds contribute omega-3 fatty acids.
- Coconut water adds hydration without excess potassium.

Preparation Time: Approximately 6 minutes.

Recipe 44: "Pomegranate Walnut Renal Revival"

Ingredients:

- 1/2 cup pomegranate seeds (low in potassium)
- 1/4 cup walnuts (source of omega-3 fatty acids)
- 1/2 cup kale leaves, stems removed (rich in vitamins)
- 1 tablespoon flaxseeds (added fiber)
- 1 cup water or unsweetened almond milk

Instructions:

- Blend pomegranate seeds, walnuts, and kale leaves until smooth.
- Add flaxseeds and water/almond milk. Blend until well combined.
- Pour into a glass and relish the renal revival with pomegranate and walnut.

Health Benefits:

- Pomegranate seeds are low in potassium and rich in antioxidants.
- Walnuts provide omega-3 fatty acids for heart health.
- Kale offers essential vitamins without excess potassium.

Preparation Time: Approximately 7 minutes.

Recipe 45: "Mango Mint Kidney Elixir"

Ingredients:

- 1 cup mango chunks (low in potassium)
- 1/4 cup fresh mint leaves (soothes digestion)
- 1/2 cup spinach leaves (rich in iron)
- 1 tablespoon hemp seeds (added omega-3 fatty acids)
- 1 cup water or coconut water

Instructions:

- Blend mango chunks, fresh mint leaves, and spinach leaves until smooth.
- Add hemp seeds and water/coconut water. Blend until well combined.
- Pour into a glass and savor the kidney elixir with mango and mint.

Health Benefits:

- Mango and spinach are low in potassium, suitable for renal diets.
- Mint soothes digestion, and hemp seeds contribute omega-3 fatty acids.
- Coconut water adds hydration without excess potassium.

Preparation Time: Approximately 5 minutes.

CONCLUSION

The Diabetic Renal Smoothie Cookbook emerges not merely as a culinary guide but as a compass for those navigating the delicate intersection of diabetes and compromised kidney function. Its emphasis on kidney-friendly fruits, vegetables, and additives reflects a thoughtful approach, acknowledging the nuanced dietary needs of individuals.

With a 10-step roadmap, it transforms smoothie creation into a personalized journey, allowing users to savor not only the flavors but also the therapeutic benefits tailored for their health.

By unraveling the unique nutritional contributions of each ingredient, this cookbook becomes a beacon for those seeking to optimize their well-being, harmonizing the science of nutrition with the art of creating flavorful, kidney-conscious smoothies.

As each sip becomes a step toward balanced nutrition and improved health, this cookbook stands as a valuable resource, offering not just recipes but a holistic approach to nourishing the body, managing diabetes, and supporting kidney health.

Elevate your wellness journey with the Diabetic Renal Smoothie Cookbook – where every blend is a deliberate and delicious step toward a healthier, happier you.

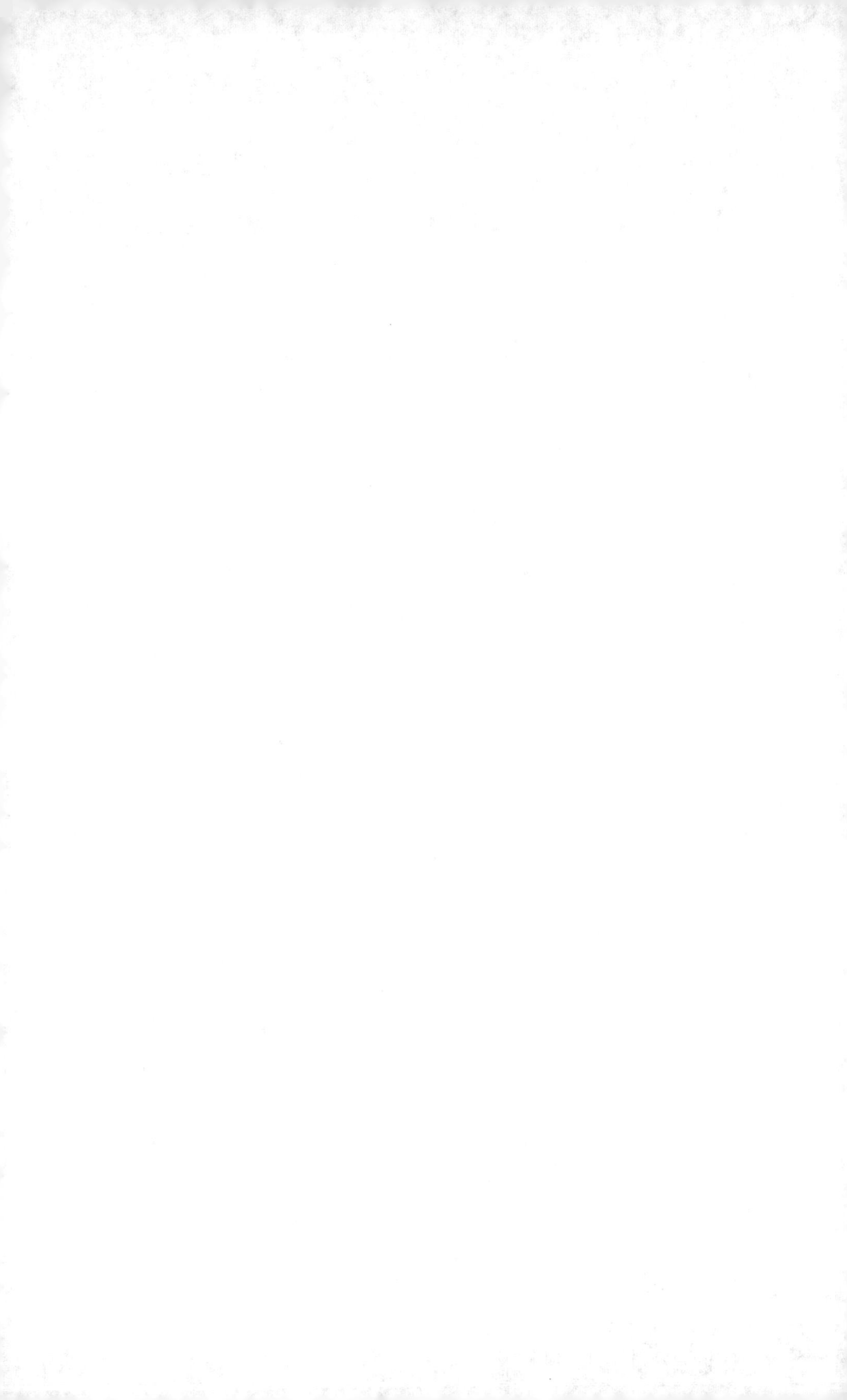